I0082479

Ketogenic Diet

Step By Step Guide And 70+ Low Carb, Proven Recipes For Rapid Weight Loss

© **Copyright 2017 By John Carter - All rights reserved.**

The contents of this book may not be reproduced, duplicated or transmitted without direct written permission from the author.

Under no circumstances will any legal responsibility or blame be held against the publisher for any reparation, damages, or monetary loss due to the information herein, either directly or indirectly.

Legal Notice:

This book is copyright protected. This is only for personal use. You cannot amend, distribute, sell, use, quote or paraphrase any part or the content within this book without the consent of the author.

Disclaimer Notice:

Please note the information contained within this document is for educational and entertainment purposes only. Every attempt has been made to provide accurate, up to date and reliable complete information. No warranties of any kind are expressed or implied. Readers acknowledge that the author is not engaging in the rendering of legal, financial, medical or professional advice. The content of this book has been derived from various sources. Please consult a licensed professional before attempting any techniques outlined in this book.

By reading this document, the reader agrees that under no circumstances are is the author responsible for any losses, direct or indirect, which are incurred as a result of the use of information contained within this document, including, but not limited to, —errors, omissions, or inaccuracies.

Bonus: FREE Report Reveals The Secrets To Lose Weight

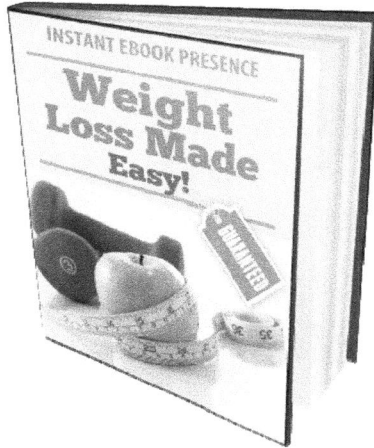

Weight loss doesn't happen from dieting only. Diets are short term solutions to shed extra weight. Diets do not work in the long term because people hate being on a diet (it's ok, you can admit that here). The only long term solution for permanent weight loss is to create new eating habits. This doesn't mean that chocolate will never pass your lips again, but it does mean looking after yourself and watching what you eat...

You can lose weight when you have the right reasons and motivation, and a part of this guide is to help you to find the motivation you need to change your weight...

Table of Contents

Introduction

All of us have too much to do and too little time. In the process of getting everything done, we often lose focus on the more important aspects of our life. One of these is probably the one thing that you should pay the most attention to, namely, health.

Being healthy is crucial to living a happy and fulfilling life. If your body is not treated right, you will soon have to face the ramifications. Just by making a few better choices in your daily life, you will see the difference it makes to everything. Just because you're always in a rush does not mean you have to skip meals or eat just anything that you can get your hands on.

Food is important for your body and the right kind of food will do you a world of good. You do not have to make any drastic changes in your diet or starve yourself either. There are a lot of fad diets and methods that claim to help you lose weight fast or get healthier than ever. Learn more about what is good for your body and what is actually going to harm you. We'll help you out with one such diet that actually works and will help you work steadily towards a healthier body.

Here you will learn all about the ketogenic diet. You might already have heard of it but may not know what it entails. We will tell you all you need to know about what it is and how it helps you. Stop following random fads that do not work or that harm your body.

As you read on, you will understand exactly why a lot of people vouch for this particular diet. You will soon be a follower as well.

Chapter 1: What Is The Ketogenic Diet?

The ketogenic or keto diet has gained quite a bit of popularity over that past few years. It is basically a diet that is quite low in carbohydrate and high in fats. The diet will help you lower blood sugar as well as insulin levels in the body. Your body's metabolism will focus on fats instead of carbohydrates for providing the energy it needs.

The ketones produced in your liver will be used for providing energy to your body. The carbohydrate intake is reduced drastically and replaced with fat. This forces your body to go into a state of ketosis. In turn, your body becomes much more efficient at burning fat and using it for energy instead of depending on carbohydrates. The fat in the liver is also converted to ketones which supply the brain with energy.

We will explain how it works further. Eating a high carbohydrate diet will make your body produce more of glucose and insulin. Since glucose is the easiest molecule to break down, the body chooses to use it as a source of energy instead of any fat that you eat. This forces the fat to get stored and makes you gain weight. However, now that you reduce the intake of carbohydrates, your body is forced to undergo ketosis. It is a natural mechanism of the body wherein the fats in the liver are broken down to produce ketones. This metabolic state is what helps you use the stored fat in your body as the main source of energy now.

There are different variants of the keto diet that you can follow:

✓ The standard ketogenic diet has very low carbohydrates, moderate protein content and high amount of fat.
✓ The high protein ketogenic diet has a higher amount of proteins than the standard diet.
✓ The targeted ketogenic diet involves adding carbohydrates in your diet according to your workout schedule.
✓ The cyclical ketogenic diet has a cycle where you follow the ketogenic diet for a certain number of days and then add carbs for a couple of days before switching back.

Let's take a look at how you can follow this diet. We have put together a list of food you should eat and those that should be avoided. This will help you keep track of what you eat and how to stay on the diet correctly.

You need to avoid most food which is carbohydrate based. List of food to avoid:

- Potatoes, carrots and other tubers or root vegetables.
- Processed vegetable oils
- Alcohol
- Diet or low-fat products
- Fruits
- Grains and starches like rice, pasta, cereal, etc.
- Lentils, peas, chickpeas and other beans or legumes
- Sugar-free foods

Eat food that is low carb but has enough proteins and fats. List of food to eat:

- Low carb vegetables like tomatoes and onions
- Nuts and seeds like chia seeds, almonds, flaxseeds, etc.
- Eggs
- Chicken, bacon, turkey, red meat, ham

- Grass-fed butter and cream
- Healthy oils like olive oil, coconut oil, avocado oil
- Avocados or guacamole
- Unprocessed cheese
- Salmon, trout, mackerel and other fatty fish
- Leafy greens like kale and spinach

The list of what to eat and what to avoid will help you choose your food. Stay away from anything which isn't keto friendly and you will soon see results. There are so many recipes which help you stay on this diet without it getting monotonous. You can try different keto recipes to help you prepare the right meals for your diet and to eat something delicious and new every day. When you get hungry in between meals, eat a small portion of some keto friendly food. For instance, you can eat dark chocolate, strawberries, salsa and guacamole, boiled eggs, nuts, cheese or some yogurt.

The diet does not require you to starve yourself or give up all the food that you like. You just need to cut out a few things that you might normally eat and eat some other foods instead. If you are worried about eating out, we can help you as well. If you order a burger, don't eat the bun. Choose a meat or fish main course. Dessert can be some berries and cream or cheeses. Egg-based dishes are also a good choice. It isn't actually that hard once you stick to the basics whether it is at home or while eating at a restaurant. The changes you make on this diet are easy to maintain and show you results soon enough.

Once you start the diet, just be aware of a few things to avoid any problems.

Precautions:

✓ Keto flu is seen to occur in some people when they start the diet. The symptoms include low energy levels, sleeping problems, nausea and increased hunger pangs. It passes after a couple of weeks. You can start by reducing the carbs little by little instead of totally cutting them out of your diet.

✓ The water and mineral content in your body is affected as well so add more salt and supplements to your diet to help balance this.

✓ Eat your meals until you are full and do not try to eat less while on this diet just to lose weight faster.

✓ Certain supplements like whey, caffeine and creatine can help you ease into the diet.

The ketogenic diet is a great option for most people and is shown to be highly effective. However, if you are suffering from certain diseases or ailments, it is advised that you consult your doctor first. Making dietary changes can affect your treatment and body as well. If they say it is okay, then go ahead with it. The diet is effective if you follow it properly and consistently for some time. It won't show results in a day or two but will have long lasting effects that you will benefit from.

Chapter 2: How Does The Diet Help You Stay Healthy And Why One Should Follow It?

A number of reasons can be stated to convince anyone to follow the ketogenic diet. Just about any issue like weight loss to medical treatments is dealt with using this particular diet. Thus you can say that it is a diet for everyone. We have put together a list of all the benefits you will reap by following the keto diet.

✓ Weight loss is one of the main reasons why people go on this diet. Since the body uses fat for energy, it helps in losing a lot of the weight from your body. Your insulin levels drop on this diet and this prompts more fat to be burnt and this helps you lose weight. It has been found to be even more effective than a diet where you reduce the fat consumption a lot.

✓ Diabetes is an ailment that affects a lot of people and this diet helps them as well. Excess fat in the body is linked to prediabetes as well as type-2 diabetes. Your insulin sensitivity increases a lot when you go on the ketogenic diet and this helps to deal with these conditions. You also lose a lot of weight and all this helps in treating diabetic conditions on a huge scale.

✓ Energy levels increase and you become much more productive in return. Fats are a more satisfying source of food to consume and a very effective source of energy as well. This helps in keeping you sated and energetic at the same time all day long.

✓ Brain function or focus is improved a lot. Ketones produced while on this diet will provide fuel for the brain. The blood sugar levels in your body are also balanced better. This helps in improving the concentration levels of a person on the keto diet.

- ✓ Epilepsy is one of the main advocates of the ketogenic diet. Children afflicted with epilepsy are treated by using this diet as a form of therapy. It has been found to be effective and has been used for a very long time now. With the help of the keto diet, patients can reduce the amount of medication they require and feel much better overall.
- ✓ Acne is a common problem for most people at some age or the other. The keto diet helps in lowering insulin levels and involves less sugar consumption. This is why it helps deal with acne as well.
- ✓ Cholesterol and Blood Pressure needs to be maintained in any person. The keto diet helps in increasing HDL and decreasing LDL. The loss in weight also helps to lower high blood pressure.
- ✓ Insulin resistance can cause a lot of issues. The keto diet helps in increasing insulin sensitivity and thus deals with this condition. This can help prevent diabetes.
- ✓ Heart diseases are linked to blood pressure, body fat and blood sugar levels. The keto diet aids in maintaining the right levels in the body and thus prevents heart diseases from occurring.

As you can see, there are a number of benefits to gain by following the simple ketogenic diet. These results are why a lot

Chapter 3: Breakfast Recipes

Spinach Mushroom & Feta Crust less Quiche

Serves: 3

Ingredients
- 4 oz. button mushrooms, sliced
- 5 oz. frozen spinach, thawed
- 1 clove garlic, minced
- ½ cup milk
- 2 large eggs, whisked
- 2 tablespoons parmesan, grated
- 1 oz. feta cheese
- ¼ cup mozzarella grated
- Salt & pepper to taste

Method:
1. Preheat the oven to 350 F. Press & remove the excess moisture from the spinach.
2. Place a non-stick skillet on medium heat and spray cooking spray over it. Add mushroom and garlic and sauté until gets fully cooked and become soft.
3. Grease a pie dish with cooking spray. Spread the spinach on the pie dish and layer it with sautéed mushrooms. Top it up with crumbled feta cheese.
4. Mix together Parmesan, milk and whisked eggs. Add pepper and stir.
5. Pour into the pie dish. Sprinkle mozzarella over it.
6. Place a baking sheet in the oven and put the pie dish over it and bake until golden brown.
7. Slice and serve.

Spinach Cucumber Smoothie

Ingredients:
- 2 cups spinach
- 1 cucumber (cubed)
- 1 cup coconut milk, unsweetened
- 15 drops liquid Stevia
- ½ teaspoon xanthan gum
- 2 tablespoons of MCT oil
- 8 ice cubes

Method:
1. Wash and shred the spinach leaves.
2. In the blender, add the shredded spinach leaves and cubed cucumber.
3. Pour the unsweetened coconut milk and liquid Stevia into the blender.
4. To this mixture add half teaspoon of xanthan gum and 2 tablespoons of MCT oil.
5. Add ice cubes to the blender and mix gently using a ladle.
6. Blend for 2 minutes. The spinach shreds give this drink a wonderful texture.
7. Serve immediately.

Tomato Broccoli Frittata

Serves: 3

Ingredients
- 5 eggs, whisked
- 1 tablespoon olive oil
- 1 ounce gouda cheese, crumbled
- 1 small head broccoli, chopped into small florets
- 1 medium tomato, chopped
- 1/2 teaspoon pepper powder
- 1 small avocado, peeled, pitted, sliced

Method:
1. Add eggs, broccoli, tomato, salt and pepper to a bowl and whisk well.
2. Add cheese and mix until well combined.
3. Place an ovenproof pan over medium heat. Add oil and swirl the pan so that the oil spreads.
4. Add the egg mixture and cook until the sides are slightly set.
5. Remove from heat.
6. Bake in a preheated oven at 425 degrees F for about 20-30 minutes or until golden brown.
7. Slice and serve with avocado slices.

French toast

Serves: 9

Ingredients:
For protein bread:
- 6 eggs separated
- 2 oz. cream cheese
- ½ cup egg white

For French toast:
- 1 egg
- ½ teaspoon vanilla
- ¼ cup coconut milk or almond milk
- ½ teaspoon cinnamon powder.

For syrup:
- ¼ cup butter
- ¼ cup almond milk
- ¼ cup swerve confectioners.

Method:

1. To make bread: Beat the egg whites until very stiff.
2. Add protein powder into the egg whites and mix gently. Add cream cheese and fold gently.
3. Grease a bread pan and pour the dough into it.
4. Put it in the preheated oven at 325 degrees F and bake it until golden brown.
5. Slice the bread when completely cooled down. Make 9 slices.
6. To make French toast: Put a greased skillet on medium high flame.
7. Mix 1 egg, almond milk, vanilla and cinnamon in a bowl.
8. Coat bread slices with egg whites.
9. Grill bread slices on hot skillets until golden brown. Repeat with remaining slices.
10. To make syrup: Melt butter over high heat in a saucepan. Add swerve and milk immediately. Whisk constantly until smooth. Remove from heat and cool. Store in an airtight container in the refrigerator.
11. Top French toast with syrup and serve.

Mini Santé Fe Frittata's

Serves: 4

Ingredients:
- 5 large eggs
- 1 egg white
- 4 ounces pork sausage
- 1/4 cup milk
- 1/2 cup red bell pepper, coarsely chopped in small cubes
- 1/2 cup yellow bell pepper, coarsely chopped in small cubes
- 1/4 cup pepper Jack cheese
- Salt to taste
- Pepper powder to taste
- 1 onion, sliced
- 2 tablespoons fresh cilantro, chopped

Method:
1. Place a skillet over medium heat. Add the sausages and cook until done.
2. Remove with a slotted spoon and set aside. Crumble it when it is cooled.
3. Place the skillet back on heat. Add peppers and cook until tender. Remove from heat and set aside.
4. Add eggs, egg white and milk to a bowl and whisk well.
5. Take 6 muffin cups and grease it with a little butter or oil. Add bacon to the cups. Next layer with bell peppers.
6. Next layer with the egg mixture and finally top with cheese. Stir lightly with a fork.
7. Bake in a preheated oven at 350 degrees F for about 20-30 minutes or until it browns. Remove from the oven.
8. Loosen the edges with a knife. Invert on to a plate and serve.

Kiwi Avocado Smoothie

Ingredients:
- 2 avocados
- 1/2 cup coconut milk.
- 1/2 cup kiwis
- 1 scoop whey powder, vanilla flavored
- 1 tablespoon chia seeds
- 6 drops liquid Stevia
- 1/2 cup water
- 3 ice cubes
- Cinnamon Powder (for garnish, optional)

Method:
1. Scoop the avocados and keep aside.
2. Add the avocados and half a cup of coconut milk to a blender.
3. Add half a cup of freshly cut kiwis to the mixture and 1 scoop of vanilla flavored whey protein powder. Blend for 30 seconds on medium.
4. Add the chia seeds and liquid Stevia to the mixture in the blender.
5. Pour half a cup of water and ice cubes into the blender.
6. Blend at medium speed until smooth.
7. Garnish with cinnamon powder and serve chilled.

Middle Eastern Shakshuka

Serves: 6

Ingredients:

- 18 ounces stew meat
- 5 cloves garlic, sliced
- 1 large onion, chopped
- 3 poblano peppers, chopped
- 1 large red bell pepper, chopped
- 1 large green bell pepper, chopped
- 2 bay leaves
- 1 ½ teaspoons paprika
- 1 ½ teaspoons ground cumin
- ¾ teaspoon crushed red pepper flakes
- Salt to taste
- Pepper to taste
- 3 tablespoons extra virgin olive oil
- ¾ cup tomato sauce
- 1 ½ cans (15 ounces each) diced tomatoes

Method:

1. Mix together in a large bowl, cumin, paprika, salt and pepper. Add meat and toss until well coated.
2. Heat and pan on medium flame and add oil. When the oil is heated, add beef with the spices and sauté until light brown.
3. Add onions, bell pepper, poblano pepper and garlic and sauté until onions are translucent.
4. Add bay leaves, crushed red pepper, and tomatoes with its juice and mash lightly the tomatoes. Stir well and cook on medium heat for 20 minutes.
5. Once the beef is cooked, discard the bay leaf and tomato sauce. Stir well. Taste and adjust the seasoning if necessary.
6. Make 6 cavities in the mixture. Crack an egg into each. Cover and cook for the remaining cook time or until the eggs are cooked as per your desire.

Italian Omelet

Ingredients
- 6 eggs
- 3 ounces full fat Brie cheese, sliced
- 3 tablespoons butter
- 15 Kalamata olives, pitted
- 3 tablespoons MCT oil
- 1/2 teaspoon salt
- 1 1/2 teaspoons Herbes De Provence
- 1 large avocado, peeled, pitted, cut into thick slices

Method
1. Add eggs, oil, herbes de Provence, olives and salt. Whisk well.
2. Place a nonstick skillet over medium - high heat. Add butter. When the butter melts, add avocado and fry until golden brown all over. Remove and set aside.
3. Place the skillet back on high heat. Add the egg mixture into it.
4. Place the cheese slice on the egg. Cover and cook until the underside is golden brown.
5. Flip sides and cook the other side too. Remove from the pan.
6. Slice into 6 wedges. Top with avocado slices and serve.

Keto Kale Herbs Smoothie

Ingredients
- 1 bunch kale
- 1 teaspoon salt
- 2 tablespoons collagen
- 2 teaspoons of apple cider vinegar
- 1 teaspoons of oregano powder
- 2 teaspoons butter
- 10 drops of MCT oil

Directions:
1. Take a bunch of kale and wash it clean under running water.
2. Cook in a steam cooker for about 8 minutes. Allow the kale to cool for a while.
3. Drain the water and add it to the blender.
4. Add a teaspoon of salt and a couple of tablespoons of collagen.
5. Take two tablespoons of apple cider vinegar and add it to the mixture and mix it well.
6. Now add a seasoning of a teaspoon of oregano powder. Along with the seasoning add 3 teaspoons of butter and 10 drops of MCT oil.
7. Switch on the blender and blend the ingredients for two minutes until the mixture is smooth in texture.
8. Serve immediately

Flax Sandwich Buns

Serves: 3

Ingredients
- 9 tablespoons flaxseed meal
- 1 teaspoon caraway seeds
- 2 teaspoons onion powder
- 3 large eggs
- 1 teaspoon baking powder
- 1 1/2 tablespoons water
- 2 drops Stevia
- 1 1/2 tablespoons olive oil

Method
1. Mix together all the dry ingredients in a bowl.
2. Mix together all the wet ingredients in a bowl.
3. Pour the wet ingredients into the bowl of dry ingredients and mix well.
4. Pour into greased muffin pan (Fill up to 2/3)
5. Bake in a preheated oven at 325 degrees F for about 15 minutes or until it done.
6. Slit in the middle, horizontally. Serve with toppings of your choice.

Vanilla Pumpkin Squash Smoothie

Ingredients:
- 1 medium pumpkin
- 1/2 cup whey powder, vanilla flavored
- 1 teaspoon vanilla essence
- 2 cups almond milk

Method:
1. Preheat oven to 300 degrees Fahrenheit.
2. Halve the pumpkins and keep both the halves face down in a baking tray.
3. Bake until tender (about half an hour.) Remove the pumpkin halves from the oven and insert a needle or fork to check if done.
4. Allow to cool for a few minutes.
5. Once cooled, remove seeds using a spoon.
6. Scoop out the pumpkin flesh into a big bowl.
7. Add whey powder and vanilla essence to this mixture.
8. Blend for 2 minutes at medium speed until smooth and then add in the almond milk and blend for another minute.
9. Pour into glasses and refrigerate. This smoothie can be stored for up to a week.

Eggs Baked In a Skillet

Serves: 2

Ingredients:
- 1/3 cup plain Greek yogurt
- 1 tablespoon unsalted butter, divided
- 2 tablespoons leek, chopped
- 1 clove garlic, halved
- Salt to taste
- 1 tablespoon olive oil
- 1 scallion, chopped
- 1 teaspoon fresh lemon juice
- 5 cups fresh spinach, chopped
- ½ teaspoon fresh oregano, chopped
- Crushed red pepper flakes to taste
- 2 large eggs

Method:

1. Add garlic & salt to the bowl of yogurt and set aside for some time.
2. Place a heavy skillet on medium heat. Add half the butter, when butter melts add leek and scallion.
3. Lower the heat. Sauté until it becomes tender.
4. Increase heat. Add spinach, lemon juice & salt. Sauté until spinach wilts.
5. Transfer the mixture into an ovenproof skillet. Make 2 deep cavities in the skillet.
6. Break eggs carefully in each cavity. Sprinkle salt over it. Place the skillet in a preheated oven at 300 degrees F and bake until the eggs set.
7. Place a small saucepan with remaining butter over medium low heat. Add red pepper flakes and salt. When it becomes frothy, add oregano and cook for 30 seconds and remove from heat.
8. Remove garlic from yogurt. Top the spinach & eggs with yogurt and sprinkle spiced butter over it.
9. Serve.

Taiwanese Oyster Omelet

Serves: 1

Ingredients:
- 2 ounces shelled oyster with juice
- ½ teaspoon arrowroot powder
- 1 tablespoon sweet potato starch
- 1 egg
- 2 teaspoons lard
- 2 teaspoons olive oil
- 1/8 teaspoon sesame oil
- 2 teaspoons peanut oil
- 1 tablespoon green onion, minced
- 1/3 cup baby bok Choy leaves, separated
- White pepper powder to taste
- Salt to taste

For the omelet sauce:
- ½ teaspoon ketchup
- ½ teaspoon hoisin sauce
- 1/8 teaspoon rice vinegar
- ¼ teaspoon Sriracha sauce
- ¼ teaspoon Chinese fine chili sauce

Method:

1. To make omelet sauce: Add all the ingredients of the omelet sauce into a bowl along with a teaspoon of boiling water. Stir and set aside.
2. Retain about 2 teaspoons of the liquid and drain the oysters.
3. Add sweet potato starch, arrowroot powder, salt, oyster liquid, and 1-teaspoon water into a bowl and mix well.
4. Add eggs, salt, pepper and sesame oil into another bowl and whisk well.
5. Heat a pan on medium flame. Add lard. When lard melts, add bok Choy and sauté until it wilts.
6. Pour the sauce mixture over it. Sprinkle oysters over it. Let it cook until the mixture turns transparent.
7. Pour egg mixture over it.
8. Close the lid. Cook for 2 mins under steam and then uncover and remove on a plate.
9. Garnish with green onions and serve.

Broccoli and Cheese Omelet

Serves - 2

Ingredients:
- 4 egg whites
- 2 eggs
- 1 cup broccoli, chopped into small pieces, cooked
- 2 tablespoons almond milk
- Salt to taste
- Pepper powder to taste
- 2 slices Swiss cheese
- Cooking spray

Method:
1. Add eggs, whites, milk, salt and pepper to a bowl and whisk well.
2. Place a nonstick skillet over medium heat. Spray with cooking spray.
3. When the pan is heated, add half the egg mixture. Swirl the pan so that the egg spreads.
4. Place a slice of cheese at the center of the omelet. Place half the broccoli over the cheese.
5. Cook until the egg sets. Fold the sides over the broccoli. Remove on to a plate and serve.
6. Repeat the above 3 steps with the remaining eggs and broccoli.

Chocolate Sesame Smoothie

Ingredients
- 2 scoops of low carbohydrate powdered protein
- 2 teaspoons cocoa powder, unsweetened
- 1 teaspoon husk from psyllium
- 300 ml water
- 2 tablespoons sesame oil
- 5 drops liquid sweetening agent
- 200 ml cooking cream, with no more than 35g of fat

Method:
1. Mix the protein powder, cocoa powder, and psyllium husk in a large glass.
2. To this mixture, add about 300ml water and shake well until it is smooth. (You can alternatively use a blender for the same, but works well in a glass too)
3. To this, add 2 tablespoons of sesame oil and the liquid sweetening agent. (The sesame oil provides valuable nutrients to the shake while giving it a nutty texture.)
4. Scoop the cooking cream and add it to the mixture. Do not shake but gently mix until the ingredients are homogenous.
5. Add ice cubes and consume within half an hour.

Cinnamon Muffins

Serves - 4

Ingredients

<u>For the muffins:</u>
- 1/2 cup coconut flour
- 6 eggs
- 4 tablespoons flaxseed powder
- 20 walnuts, chopped
- 1 cup plain yogurt
- 4 tablespoons almond milk
- 1/2 cup sugar free maple syrup
- 1/2 teaspoon soda
- 1/2 teaspoon salt
- 4 teaspoons ground cinnamon

<u>For the glaze:</u>
- 4 tablespoons butter, melted
- 1/2 cup sugar free maple syrup
- 4 teaspoons ground cinnamon

Method

1. To make muffins: Mix together all the dry ingredients in a bowl.
2. Mix together all the wet ingredients in a bowl.
3. Add the dry ingredients to the wet ingredients and whisk well.
4. Pour into greased muffin cups (fill up to 3/4).
5. Bake in a preheated oven at 350 degrees F for about 20-30 minutes or until it turns light brown. Remove from the oven and set aside to cool for about 10 minutes.
6. Meanwhile, mix together the ingredients of the glaze.
7. Loosen the edges with a knife. Invert on to a plate and brush with the glaze.
8. Serve warm.

Chapter 4: Soup & Salad Recipes

Spicy Thai Shrimp Salad

Serves: 6

Ingredients:
- 1 ½ pounds small shrimp, peeled, deveined
- 6 teaspoons fish sauce
- 3 tablespoons lime juice
- 1 ½ tablespoons olive oil
- Stevia drops to taste
- 1 medium red bell pepper, thinly sliced
- 1 medium yellow bell pepper, thinly sliced
- 2 medium cucumbers, thinly sliced
- Salt to taste
- ½ teaspoon red crushed pepper
- 2 tablespoons fresh basil, minced
- 2 tablespoons fresh mint, minced
- 2 tablespoons fresh cilantro, minced

Method:
1. Sauté the shrimp on medium heat for about 2 mins until they get cooked.
2. You can even just steam them if you prefer it that way.
3. Transfer the shrimp to a bowl. Add rest of the ingredients and mix well.
4. Serve!

Chicken Salad Stuffed Avocado

Serves 2:

Ingredients:
- 6 oz. chicken breast
- 2 tablespoon diced onions
- 2 avocadoes
- 2 stalk celery
- 2/3 cup sour cream
- Salt and pepper as per taste

Method:
1. On low heat cook the chicken breast until it gets tender. Shred the chicken with help of forks.
2. In a bowl mix chicken, red onion and celery.
3. Cut & scoop out some avocado and add in the chicken mixture.
4. Mix the sour cream and add salt & pepper.
5. Fill the avocado halves with the mixture and serve.

Strawberry Zoodle Salad with Goat cheese and Pistachios

Serves 2

Ingredients:
For the salad:
- 2 strawberries, sliced
- 2 cups zucchini noodles
- 2 tablespoons herbed goat cheese, sliced and crumbled
- 2 tablespoons pistachios

For dressing:
- 8 strawberries
- 4 tablespoons avocado oil
- 4 tablespoons balsamic vinegar
- 1 teaspoon garlic, minced
- ¼ teaspoon salt
- ¼ teaspoon freshly cracked pepper

Method:
1. Mix salad ingredients in a bowl.
2. Place dressing ingredients in a blender and blend until well combined.
3. Toss the salad with 2 tablespoon of strawberry balsamic dressing and serve.

Salmon Salad

Serves: 4

Ingredients:
- 3 stalks celery, thinly sliced
- 2 shallots, minced
- 2 cloves of garlic, minced
- 1 bell pepper, thinly sliced
- 1 medium cucumber
- ½ pint tomatoes
- ¼ olive oil or to taste
- Juice of ½ a lemon
- Zest of ½ a lemon
- 1 tablespoon red wine vinegar
- ½ teaspoon kosher salt or to taste
- ½ teaspoon fresh or dried dill
- ¼ teaspoon freshly ground black pepper
- ¼ teaspoon smoked paprika
- ¼ teaspoon ground cumin
- ¼ teaspoon crushed red pepper flakes
- 2 cans salmon, drained

Method:
1. Halve the cucumber lengthwise and then slice it. Halve the tomatoes.
2. Add all the ingredients to a large bowl. Toss well and refrigerate for an hour.
3. Add more seasoning if necessary and serve.

Spinach and Bacon Salad

Serves: 3

Ingredients:
- 4 cups raw spinach
- ½ cup chopped shallots
- 6 slices bacon
- 1 tbsp. butter

Method:
1. First slice the bacon strips finely. Melt butter on a skillet placed on medium flame.
2. Add the shallots and the bacon to the skillet. Sauté until the shallots have turned golden brown and are translucent.
3. Now, add the spinach and cook until the leaves have wilted. Toss the ingredients and serve hot.

Thai Style Chicken Salad

Serves: 3

Ingredients:
- 1 shallot, minced
- 3 tablespoons mayonnaise
- 3 tablespoons nonfat plain yogurt
- 1 teaspoon lemon juice
- 1 tablespoon chili sauce
- 3 cups chicken, skinless, boneless, chopped
- 1 teaspoon lemon juice
- Pepper powder to taste
- Salt to taste
- 1 small red bell pepper, chopped
- ½ cup Napa cabbage, thinly sliced
- 2 tablespoons cashews, chopped, toasted
- 1-tablespoon peanut oil.

Method:
1. Stir-fry the chicken on medium heat using some peanut oil.
2. Mix the rest of the ingredients and toss the stir-fried chicken in it.
3. Serve.

Chicken, Tomato and Bacon Salad

Ingredients

For the Salad

- 2 large uncooked chicken breasts (cut them into chunks that are one inch each)
- 4 tsp. Canadian Steak Brand (you could use any brand that you want)
- 4 tbsp. butter
- 10 slices bacon
- 2 small tomatoes
- 3 ounces Muenster cheese

For the dressing

- 3 tbsp. butter
- 2 raw eggs (preferably eggs from a pastured chicken. This egg will be richer)
- 3 ounces mayonnaise
- 3 tsp. lemon juice
- 1 tsp. salt

Method

The Salad

1. Add the Canadian steak seasoning to the chicken and spread it neatly.
2. Take a pan and place it on a medium flame and add the butter. When the butter begins to melt, add the chicken breasts and sauté it.
3. Make sure that it is cooked through before you remove it off the pan. Leave it aside to cool down to room temperature.
4. Cut the bacon into thin strips. Sauté the strips in a pan on a medium flame until you drain all the oil.

The Dressing

1. Take a small pan and add the butter to it. Place the pan on low heat. Once the butter melts pull the pan off the flame and leave the butter to cool.
2. Add the yolk to the butter and whisk the two well until the mixture has become glossy and smooth.
3. Add the remaining ingredients and whisk until the mixture is smooth.

The finished Salad

1. Take a plate and add all the ingredients and the dressing and mix them well.
2. Ensure that the ingredients are coated well with the dressing.

Coconut Lime Chicken & Snow Peas Salad

Serves: 4

Ingredients:
- 16 ounces chicken tenders
- 2 cups light coconut milk
- Stevia drops to taste
- ½ cup lime juice
- 8 romaine lettuce, shredded
- 2 cups snow peas, sliced
- 2 cups red cabbage, shredded
- ¼ cup red onion, minced
- 1/3 cup fresh cilantro, chopped
- 1 teaspoon salt or to taste

Method:
1. Whisk together in a large bowl, coconut milk, Stevia, lime juice, and salt. Pour ¾ of it into a bowl.
2. Add chicken and stir.
3. Let it sit for 30 mins and then transfer the mix to a pan. Cook the chicken in the same juice on a medium flame. Allow it to soak in most of the juices as it cooks.
4. Remove the chicken with a slotted spoon. When cool enough to handle, slice the chicken.
5. Add vegetables into the large dish, which has ¼ the dressing. Toss well.
6. Divide and place the salad on individual serving plates. Place the chicken slices over it. Ladle a little of the cooked liquid over it and serve.

Lobster Salad

Serves: 4

Ingredients:
- 1 1/2 pounds Northern lobster (steamed)
- 4 cup Chinese cabbage (Bok-Choy or Pak-Choi), shredded
- 1 small red peppers
- 8 medium spring onions
- 2 tablespoons sesame seeds
- Salt to taste
- Pepper powder to taste

For the dressing:
- 4 tablespoons rice vinegar
- 4 tablespoons tamari sauce
- 2 tablespoons canola oil
- 2 teaspoons sesame oil
- 2 teaspoons ginger, minced

Method:
1. To make the dressing: Mix together all the ingredients of the dressing in jar and shake vigorously.
2. Mix together rest of the ingredients in a large bowl. Pour dressing over the salad. Toss well and serve.

Cream of Broccoli Soup

Serves 3

Ingredients:
- 1 red onion, chopped chunky
- ½ teaspoon tamari sauce
- 1 tablespoon coconut oil
- 2.5 cup of water
- 1 cup of fresh Broccoli florets
- ½ tablespoon Chicken soup powder
- ½ cup of whipping cream.

Method:
1. Heat coconut oil in a pan and sauté red onions in it.
2. Add broccoli and water. Cook for 10 minutes.
3. Put the soup in a blender and make puree.
4. Lower the heat and add cream. Stir
5. Serve hot in soup bowls.

Thai Hot and Sour Shrimp Soup

Serves: 2

Ingredients:

- 8 to 10 shrimp, peeled, with its tail on, and deveined, set aside the shells
- 1 small onion, chopped
- 1 tablespoon coconut oil, divided
- 1 inch piece galangal, peeled, chopped into thick slices
- 2 cloves garlic
- 2 fresh kaffir leaves or ¼ teaspoon lemon zest, grated
- 1 stalk lemon grass, chopped into 1 inch pieces
- 1 Thai red chili, roughly chopped
- ¼ pound crimini or shiitake or oyster or button mushrooms, rinsed, sliced into wedges
- 2 ½ cups chicken broth
- 1 tablespoon fresh lime juice
- ½ small green zucchini, sliced
- Salt to taste
- Pepper to taste
- 1 tablespoon fish sauce
- 1 tablespoon fresh lime juice
- 2 tablespoons fresh basil, chopped
- 2 tablespoons fresh cilantro, chopped
- Salt to taste
- Pepper to taste

Method:

1. Heat a pan on medium flame. Add ½ tablespoon coconut oil. When the oil is heated, add shrimp shells that were kept aside and stir constantly until they turn red in color.
2. Add onions, galangal, garlic, lemon grass, kaffir lime leaves or fresh lime zest, Thai red chili, salt and pepper. Sauté for a few minutes until the onions turn translucent.
3. Add broth and stir.
4. Let the mix cook for 10 mins or until everything gets well incorporated and cooked.
5. Remove the shrimp shells with a slotted spoon. Discard the shells.
6. Transfer the stock into a bowl and set aside.
7. Add the remaining coconut oil into a pot.
8. When the oil is heated, add zucchini slices and mushroom and season with salt and pepper. Sauté for a few minutes until tender.
9. Add the cooked broth into the pot. Add shrimp into the pot and stir. Let it cook for another 5 – 7 minutes.
10. Add lime juice, salt, pepper, and fish sauce. Stir well. Taste and adjust the seasoning if necessary.
11. Simmer for a couple of minutes or until the shrimp is cooked. Add fresh cilantro and basil and stir.
12. Ladle into soup bowls and serve immediately.

Mallow Soup

Serves: 3

Ingredients:
- 3 cups water
- 3 pieces chicken, bite sized
- 1 chicken bouillon cube
- 1 small onion, chopped
- 1 package (14 ounces) frozen Moulkhia, minced or chopped
- ½ teaspoon ground allspice
- 2 cloves garlic
- 2 tablespoons olive oil

Method:
1. Heat the oil in a pan and sauté the onions in it. When the onions turn translucent, ass the chicken and stir. Add the water and let it cook
2. Once the chicken is cooked, let it sit for a while. Discard the fat that is floating on the top.
3. Add moulkia, bouillon cubes, allspice and salt and let the mix simmer for about 10 minutes.
4. Meanwhile, smash together garlic and little salt.
5. Place a small pan over medium heat. Add oil into it. When the oil is heated, add garlic and sauté until golden brown. Transfer the chicken mix to this oil and garlic mix and let it simmer for another 5 mins.
6. Ladle into soup bowls and serve hot.

Chicken Zoodle Soup (instant pot recipe)

Serves: 4 cups

Ingredients:
- 1 small onion, chopped
- 2 teaspoons coconut oil
- 2 cloves garlic, minced
- 1 jalapeño, chopped
- 1 small red bell pepper, thinly sliced
- ½ pound chicken breasts, thinly sliced against the grain
- 3 cups chicken broth
- 1 tablespoon fish sauce
- Juice of a lime
- 1 medium zucchini
- 8 ounces full fat coconut milk
- 2 teaspoons Thai green curry paste
- ¼ cup fresh cilantro

Method:
1. Select 'Sauté' option. Add oil. When the oil is melted, add onions and sauté until translucent.
2. Add jalapeño, green curry paste and garlic and sauté until fragrant. Add broth and coconut milk and whisk well.
3. Add red bell pepper, chicken, and fish sauce and stir. Press 'Cancel' button.
4. Select 'Soup' option and timer for 15 minutes. Let the pressure release naturally. Add cilantro and lemon juice and stir.
5. Meanwhile make the zoodles as follows: Make noodles of the zucchini using a spiralizer. Alternately, use a julienne peeler and make the noodles.
6. Divide and place the zoodles into 4 cups. Pour the soup into it. Serve immediately.

Cream of Mushroom Soup

Serves 3:

Ingredients:
- 1 onion, chopped into chunks
- ½ tablespoon tamari sauce
- 1 tablespoon coconut oil
- 1 packet of Portabella Mushroom
- ½ cup of whipping cream
- 2.5 cup of water
- ½ tablespoon of Mushroom Soup powder

Method:
1. Heat coconut oil in a pan and add onions and sauté until translucent.
2. Add Portabella mushrooms and tamari sauce and cook for 2 minutes
3. Pour water and cook until tender.
4. Put the soup in a blender and puree it.
5. Pour soup back into the pan. Heat the soup.
6. Lower the heat and add whipping cream into it. Stir.
7. Pour in soup bowls and serve hot.

Chapter 5: Snack Recipes

Keto Italian Meatballs

Serves: 4

Ingredients

- 4 ounces minced white onion
- 2 tsp. Italian seasoning
- 1.5 tsp. sea salt
- 1 tsp. freshly ground black pepper
- 1 cup shredded Romano / parmesan /asiago mix
- 1 large eggs
- 1 pound ground beef (92% lean)
- 1 cup cold whole milk ricotta cheese
- 1 tbsp. olive oil
- 1.5 tsp. granulated garlic

Method

1. Preheat the oven to 350 degrees F.
2. Take a saucepan and place it on medium flame. Add the olive to the pan. Once the oil has heated, add the onions and sauté until they are translucent.
3. Once the onions have turned translucent, take the pan off the flame and leave the onions to cool.
4. Mince the Romano/ parmesan/ asiago mix in a blender or a food processor.
5. Take a large mixing bowl and add the eggs and the ricotta cheese to the bowl and mix well! Make sure that there are no lumps in the mixture and that it is smooth.
6. Add the salt, pepper and the remaining spices to the mixture and stir well. Ensure that the spices and the egg mixture have blended well.
7. Add the sautéed onions to the egg mixture along with the minced Romano / Parmesan / asiago mix. Add the ingredients well.
8. Add vinegar to the bowl and ensure that the mixture is smooth.
9. When the mixture has blended well, add the beef to the mixture. You will need to ensure that the mixture is well balanced once you add the beef to the mixture. Ensure that the taste is balanced throughout the mixture!
10. Divide the entire mixture in portions with one ounce each. You will have 20 sized pieces of the beef.
11. You will need to make a ball out of the 20 pieces that you make.
12. Grease a cookie sheet well with the olive oil and place the beef meatballs on the tray. Place the tray in the oven for twenty minutes! Make sure that they are brown on the outside before you serve them!

Chicken and cheese enchilada

Serves: 3

Ingredients:
- 3 cups mixed vegetables
- 2 lb. ground chicken
- 1 cup melted cheese
- ½ cup chopped shallots
- 2 tortillas
- 1 tbsp. butter

Method:
- Melt butter on a skillet placed on medium flame.
- Add the shallots and chicken to the skillet. Sauté until the shallots have turned golden brown and are translucent.
- Toss the ingredients.
- Transfer this mixture onto the toruntila and roll it. Add the molten cheese.
- Serve with a mayonnaise dip.

Chinese Five Spice Chicken

Serves: 8

Ingredients
- 1 ½ pounds chicken leg quarters
- 2 cloves garlic, minced
- 1 inch piece ginger, grated
- 2 teaspoons five spice powder
- 1 medium onion, finely chopped
- 2 tablespoons fresh cilantro
- ½ cup chicken broth
- Salt to taste
- Pepper to taste

Method:
1. Place the chicken legs in a pot. Pour the broth over it. Sprinkle, garlic, ginger and onions over it. Finally sprinkle five-spice powder, salt and pepper.
2. Let the mixture simmer until it gets well cooked.
3. Serve hot.

Cheddar Pepper Biscuits

Serves: 6

Ingredients
- 5 cups almond flour
- 12 ounces Colby jack cheese (shredded)
- 10 tbsp. butter
- 16 ounces cream cheese
- 4 large eggs or 6 medium eggs
- 4 tsp. ground pepper
- 2 tsp. baking soda
- 2 tsp. Xanthan gum
- 2 tsp. sea salt

Method

1. Take a cookie sheet and grease it well. Line it with parchment paper if you do not want to grease it.
2. Then preheat the oven to 300 degrees Fahrenheit.
3. Process the shredded cheese and one cup of the almond flour in a food processor until they have blended well and are granular. Keep this aside.
4. Take a large mixing bowl. Add the butter and the cream cheese to the bowl and place. You have to melt the better a little. Once it has melted, mix the butter and the cheese together. Make sure that the mixture is smooth and glossy.
5. Add the eggs to the mixture and continue to whisk. Make sure that the mixture is smooth and glossy.
6. Add the pepper, the Xanthan gum, baking soda and the salt to the mixture.
7. Add the remaining almond flour and cheese mixture to the egg mixture and whisk well.
8. Once the ingredients have blended well, add the almond flour that is left and continue to fold the mixture well. You have to ensure that the dough has formed.
9. Take a tablespoon and scoop the dough and place it on the cookie sheet. Keep the cookies one inch apart. If you want you could flatten the dough a little to ensure that you have a smooth biscuit.
10. Place the cookie sheet in the oven and bake for thirty minutes. You will need to leave the biscuits in until they have a golden brown color.
11. Remove the biscuits from the oven and cool to room temperature. You can serve it with a glass of milk.

Taco Bites

Serves: 3

Ingredients
- 1 tbsp. butter
- ½ yellow onion (chopped)
- 1.5 cloves garlic (minced)
- ½ pound beef (ground)
- 2 ounces can green chilies
- 1 tsp. cumin (ground)
- 1tsp. chili powder
- ½ tsp. coriander (ground)
- ½ cup sour cream
- 1 cup Cheddar Cheese (grated)

Method
1. Preheat the oven to 350 degrees Fahrenheit.
2. Take a medium skillet and place it on a medium flame. Add the butter to the skillet and wait until the butter melts.
3. Add the onions to the skillet and sauté. Make sure that they have become soft.
4. Add the beef to the skillet and cook until it is brown.
5. Add the spices to the skillet along with the green chilies from the pan and cook for five minutes.
6. Reduce the heat and add the cheese and the cream to the skillet and simmer for a few minutes.
7. Continue to stir the mixture for a few minutes until the cheese has melted and has mixed well into the beef.
8. Pre bake some piecrusts and add the mixture to the crusts.
9. Bake the crusts in the oven with the beef for a few minutes until the cheese is bubbling.

Coconut Fruity Smoothie

Ingredients
- 8 ice cubes
- 3/4 cup coconut milk, unsweetened
- 1/4 cup heavy cream
- 15 drops liquid Stevia
- 1/2 teaspoon mango extract
- 1/4 teaspoon banana extract
- 1/4-teaspoon blueberry extract.
- 2 tablespoons flaxseed oil
- 1 tablespoon MCT oil

Method:
1. Pour the ice cubes in a blender. Add the coconut milk and heavy cream to the ice cubes.
2. To this mixture add 15 drops of liquid Stevia. Mix well and add half a teaspoon of mango extract and a quarter teaspoon of each blueberry and banana extract.
3. Blend at medium speed for 2 minutes and let it stand for 30 seconds.
4. Then add in the flaxseed oil and MCT oil and blend for another minute
5. Pour into glasses and serve chilled.

Zucchini Pancakes

Serves: 3

Ingredients
- 2 Zucchinis (shredded)
- 2 cups almond flour
- 3 eggs
- 2 tsp. dried basil
- 2 tsp. dried parsley
- Salt and Pepper to taste
- 3 tbsp. Butter

Method
1. Take a small mixing bowl and add the shredded zucchini, along with the basil and the almond flour.
2. Mix the ingredients well. Once the zucchini is coated well with the flour, add the parsley, pepper and the salt to the bowl.
3. Ensure that the taste of the mixture is well balanced.
4. You can make close to 10 patties from the mixture that you have just made.
5. Take a large non – stick sauce pan and place it on a medium flame.
6. Add one teaspoon to the pan. Once the butter has started warming up, add the patties and cook them one after the other.
7. Ensure that you remove the patty off the pan when it is brown on both sides.

Tandoori Chicken

Serves: 6

Ingredients:
- 1 teaspoon garlic paste
- 1 teaspoon ginger paste
- 6 bone-in chicken thighs, skinless, trimmed of fat
- 1 teaspoon ground cumin
- 1 teaspoon salt
- ½ teaspoon ground cinnamon
- 1 teaspoon ground turmeric
- ¼ teaspoon ground cloves
- ½ cup thick yogurt
- 2 tablespoons fresh lemon juice
- 2 tablespoons fresh cilantro, chopped
- Onion rings to serve (optional)

Method:

1. To get thick yogurt, place yogurt in a fine mesh strainer for about an hour. The excess liquid will get drained.
2. Mix together in a bowl all the ingredients except chicken, lemon juice, and cilantro.
3. Add chicken and mix until well coated. Cover and refrigerate for at least 2-3 hours.
4. Remove from the refrigerator at least 30 minutes before cooking.
5. Heat a pan with little oil and shallow fry the tandoori chicken until it's done from all sides (approximately 2-3 minutes each side)
6. Alternately, you can also bake them in an over. Preheat the oven at 300 degrees F for 30 mins. Place the marinated chicken pieces on a baking tray. Let it bake for about 30 minutes at the same heat.
7. Transfer on to a serving plate. Sprinkle lemon juice and cilantro over it. Serve with onion rings if desired.

Bacon burritos

Serves: 3

Ingredients:
- 4 cups raw spinach
- ½ cup chopped shallots
- 6 slices bacon
- 2 tortillas
- 1 tbsp. butter

Method:
1. First slice the bacon strips finely. Melt butter on a skillet placed on medium flame.
2. Add the shallots and the bacon to the skillet. Sauté until the shallots have turned golden brown and are translucent.
3. Now, add the spinach and cook until the leaves have wilted.
4. Toss the ingredients.
5. Transfer this mixture onto the tortilla and roll it.
6. Serve with a mayonnaise dip.

Dragon Fruit Coconut Smoothie

Ingredients:
- ½ dragon fruit (coarsely chopped)
- 1/2 cup mixed Galia melon
- 1/2 cup coconut milk
- 2 scoops whey protein powder, vanilla flavored
- 1 tablespoon chia seeds
- 6 to 8 drops of liquid Stevia (recipe says half a dozen)
- 1/2 cup water
- 4 ice cubes

Method:
1. In a blender, add the chopped dragon fruit and Galia melon. Pour half a cup of coconut milk and 2 scoops of whey protein powder into the blender.
2. To this mixture add a tablespoon of chia seeds and 6 to 8 drops of liquid Stevia extract.
3. Pour the water and add the ice cubes.
4. Set the blender on medium setting and blend the ingredients until the mixture is smooth in texture.
5. Pour into glasses. Serve immediately.

Crab meat bites

Serves: 2

Ingredients
- ½ can crab meat
- 4 ounces cream cheese
- ¼ cup cream
- ½ tbsp. lemon juice
- 1 tbsp. onion (finely chopped)
- 1 tbsp. red bell pepper (finely chopped)
- 1 tbsp. celery (finely chopped)
- ¼ cup mustard (dry)
- ¼ tsp. salt

Method
1. Preheat the oven to 350 degrees Fahrenheit.
2. Drain the crabmeat from the can and clean the meat well. Remove any bits of shell.
3. Make sure that the cream cheese is left to soften at the room temperature.
4. Take a large mixing bowl and add the ingredients to the bowl.
5. Bake miniature tarts in the oven.
6. Add the crab mixture to the tarts and place them in the oven for ten minutes at 350 degrees F. Serve hot.

Lebanese Spiced Mushrooms (Instant pot recipe)

Serves: 2

Ingredients:
- 6 ounces mushrooms, cut into thick slices
- 1 teaspoon fresh mint, chopped
- 2 teaspoons fresh parsley, chopped
- ¼ teaspoon ground cinnamon
- ¾ teaspoon ground coriander
- A pinch ground cloves
- 2 teaspoons lemon juice
- Salt to taste
- Pepper powder to taste
- 1 ½ tablespoons olive oil

Method:
1. Select 'Sauté' option. Add oil. When the oil is tender, add mushrooms, ground cloves, ground coriander and ground cinnamon.
2. Sauté for a few minutes until tender.
3. Add mint, parsley, salt, pepper and lemon juice. Toss well.
4. Serve hot.

Chapter 6: Meal Recipes

Beef and mixed vegetable Stir Fry

Serves: 4

Ingredients
- 1 lb. beef
- 2 tbsp. coconut oil
- 1 cup onion minced
- 2 cups broccoli chopped
- 1 tbsp. sesame seeds
- 3 tbsp. green onion chopped
- 1 cup chestnuts sliced

Method
1. First, clean the beef and cut it into small pieces of equal size.
2. Place a pan over medium flame. Add the coconut oil to the pan and wait for it to heat.
3. Once the coconut oil is hot, you will need to put the beef in the pan.
4. Cook the beef and make sure that it is brown on all sides.
5. Remove the beef from the pan and set it aside.
6. Add the onion and the broccoli to the pan and sauté for a few minutes. You need to make sure that the onion is translucent and that the broccoli begins to wilt.
7. Add the beef to the pan and fry for a few minutes. Once the flavors bend together. You could add more vegetables to the dish if you like.

Stuffed Chicken

Serves: 2

Ingredients:
- 4 boneless and skinless chicken breast
- ½ bottle garlic and herb marinade
- Fresh basil leaves
- 2 tomatoes (sliced)
- 4 slices mozzarella cheese
- 12 slices bacon

Method:
1. Slice chicken breast horizontally and pour marinade over chicken with breasts opened
2. Let it sit for 30 minutes
3. In the meantime, preheat oven to 400 degrees F
4. Place chicken into pan and cover the chicken with enough tomatoes
5. Place cheese on chicken and fold the chicken over and hold with toothpick
6. Wrap 3 slices bacon around each breast
7. Cook for 20 minutes
8. Turn and cook chicken for 15 more minutes

Spaghetti Squash Lasagna with Meatballs

Serves: 8

Ingredients:
- 5 cups roasted spaghetti squash (about 3)
- 2 cups parmesan cheese, grated
- 4 cups mozzarella cheese, shredded
- 2 pounds ground beef
- 1 teaspoon basil
- 2 teaspoon chili powder
- 1 teaspoon oregano
- 6 cloves garlic, peeled
- Sea salt to taste
- Pepper powder to taste
- 2 teaspoons red pepper flakes
- 3 cups low carb marinara sauce
- 2 eggs
- 2 tablespoons ghee or coconut oil

Method:

1. Preheat the oven to 350 F.
2. Peel spaghetti squash (about 3 medium sized), deseed it and chop into chunks. Roast it in the oven at 350 degrees F for about an hour. Then measure 5 cups of spaghetti squash and mash it slightly. Or you can roast the squash without chopping it. Peel, deseed and mash after roasting it.
3. Mince garlic and set aside
4. Add marinara sauce and red pepper flakes to a pan, cover and simmer for 5 minutes.
5. To make meat balls: Add ground beef, basil, chili powder, garlic, oregano, salt, pepper, and eggs to large bowl and mix well using your hands.
6. Make small meatballs of the mixture with moistened hands.
7. Place a frying pan over medium heat. Add about a tablespoon of ghee. When ghee melts, add around half the meatballs (do not crowd, fry it in batches).
8. Flip sides and cook on all sides until brown. Remove the meatballs and set aside on a plate.
9. Repeat with the remaining meatballs.
10. Take a baking dish. Spread about ¾ cup marinara sauce. Next spread half the spaghetti squash over it followed by few meatballs.
11. Next layer with Parmesan cheese followed by another layer of sauce followed by spaghetti squash.
12. Next place a few meatballs. Sprinkle half the mozzarella cheese over it. Finally layer with the remaining sauce followed by spaghetti squash, meatballs and finally mozzarella cheese.
13. Bake in a preheated oven at 350 for 30 minutes.

Kebab Chicken

Serves: 4

Ingredients:
- Almonds (handful)
- 6 jalapeno peppers (chopped and seeded)
- 8 cloves of garlic
- 1 cup fresh cilantro (chopped)
- Pinch of salt
- Juice of one lemon
- ½ cup heavy cream
- 2 pounds chicken breast (skinless & boneless)
- Butter

Method:
1. Cut chicken breast into 1 ½ inch pieces
2. Then blend almond, pepper, garlic and cilantro until smooth, once done, blend the cream. Coat the chicken with this sauce.
3. Preheat grill for 375 degrees F for 30 mins
4. Skewer meat (4 per skewer) and season eat skewer accordingly
5. Brush butter onto skewer
6. Cook chicken on medium heat until done.

Tasty Beef and Liver Burger

Serves 2

Ingredients:
- 0.6 pound ground beef
- ½ teaspoon salt
- 4 ounces chicken livers
- ¾ teaspoon ground coriander
- ½ teaspoon ground black pepper
- ½ onion, peeled
- ½ teaspoon poultry seasoning

Method:
1. Mince moderately chicken liver and onion in a food processor.
2. Add ground beef and all spices in the blender and blend together in food processor. Remove on to a bowl.
3. Divide the mixture into 4 equal portions.
4. Moisten your hands and shape the mixture into patties.
5. Grill the patties until done.
6. Serve over bed of lettuce.

Cheese Stuffed Bacon Wrapped Hot Dogs

Serves: 10

Ingredients:
- 10 hot dogs
- 20 slices bacon
- 3 ounces cheddar cheese, chopped into small rectangles
- 1 teaspoon garlic powder
- 1 teaspoon onion powder
- Salt to taste
- Pepper to taste

Method:
1. Slit the hotdogs in the middle leaving the sides intact.
2. Gently insert the cheese pieces inside the slits.
3. Wrap the hot dog tightly with 2 slices of bacon. First place a slice of bacon at one end, insert a toothpick and start wrapping. Place the next slice overlapping the end of the first one. Insert tooth picks on the other end of the hot dog.
4. Sprinkle salt, pepper, onion, and garlic powder.
5. Place on the wire rack of a preheated oven.
6. Bake at 400 degrees F for about 40 minutes or until golden brown.
7. Serve with a creamy spinach dip.

Thai Chicken Noodles

Serves: 4

Ingredients:
- 1 teaspoon curry powder
- 7 ounce chicken thighs
- 2 tablespoon unsalted butter
- 2 tablespoon coconut oil
- 3 stalks spring onion, finely chopped
- 3 cloves garlic, finely chopped
- 2 eggs
- 3 ounce bean sprouts
- 7 ounce zucchini
- 2 teaspoons soy sauce
- 1 teaspoon oyster sauce
- 1/4 teaspoon white pepper powder
- 2 teaspoons lime juice
- 2 red chilies, chopped
- Salt to taste
- Pepper to taste

Method:

1. Place the chicken in a bowl. Sprinkle curry powder, a large pinch salt, and a large pinch of pepper. Keep aside.
2. Meanwhile make noodles of the zucchini using a spiralizer.
3. To prepare the sauce: Mix together in a small bowl, soy sauce, oyster sauce, and white pepper powder.
4. Place a nonstick skillet over medium heat. Add butter and add the chicken. Fry until browned. When cool enough to handle, chop into bite sized pieces.
5. In the same pan add coconut oil. Increase to high heat. Add spring onions and sauté for a couple of minutes.
6. Add garlic and sauté for a minute. Break the eggs into the skillet and make scrambled eggs. Sauté until lightly brown.
7. Add bean sprouts and the zucchini noodles. Mix well. Add sauce and mix again.
8. Cook until there is hardly any liquid left.
9. Add the chopped chicken, lime juice and the red chilies. Mix well.
10. Serve hot.

Reuben Casserole

Serves: 4

Ingredients:
- 3/4 pound corned beef, diced
- 3/4 can sauerkraut, drained
- 1 1/2 cups Swiss cheese, shredded
- 6 tablespoons mayonnaise
- 6 ounces cream cheese
- 6 tablespoons low sugar ketchup
- 2 tablespoons pickle brine or ½ teaspoon vinegar,
- 1/2 teaspoon caraway seeds

Method:
1. Heat a saucepan over low heat. Add cream cheese, mayonnaise, and ketchup. When melted add half the Swiss cheese, sauerkraut and beef. Mix until well combined and cheese is melted.
2. Remove from heat and add pickle brine. Mix well. Transfer into a greased baking dish.
3. Sprinkle with the remaining cheese and caraway seeds.
4. Bake in a preheated oven at 350 degrees F until the cheese is slightly browned.
5. Serve hot.

Ginger pork with broccoli

Serves: 4

Ingredients
- 2 tablespoons butter
- 1 pound pork chops, sliced into small chunks
- 1 teaspoon kosher salt
- 1 teaspoon garlic powder
- 1 teaspoon ginger powder
- 1 teaspoon onion powder
- 2 tablespoons lemon juice
- ½ teaspoon fish sauce
- ½ teaspoon ground pepper
- 4 cups broccoli florets
- 1 cup coconut aminos
- Some freshly chopped cilantro leaves
- 1 teaspoon red pepper flakes
- Slices of two lemon for garnish

Method

1. Melt some butter in a pan over low heat.
2. Combine garlic powder, ginger powder, onion powder, salt and pepper in a bowl.
3. Add the pork chunks to the pan and sprinkle the spice mix on top. Cook the pork for about 3-4 minutes on high flame until it is browned form both sides. Transfer into another bowl.
4. Turn the heat to low and add the coconut aminos to the pan along with some lemon juice and fish sauce. Let this sauce simmer for about 8-9 minutes on medium heat until it is thickened.
5. Steam the broccoli florets in batches over a steamer for about 5minutes. Ensure that you do not over steam the broccoli.
6. Now place the steamed broccoli florets on a large plate. Add the cooked pork chunks over the florets.
7. Now pour the sauce on top.
8. Garnish with some fresh cilantro and lemon slices on top.
9. Serve hot.

Kale with bacon, onion and garlic

Serves 2

Ingredients
- 2 large bunches of kale leaves
- 2 cups chopped onions
- 4 cloves garlic
- 6 slices raw bacon
- 4 tbsp. butter

Method
1. Take a skillet and place it on a medium flame and add butter to it.
2. Cut the bacon into small strips or pieces and add them to the skillet.
3. Cook the bacon well.
4. Add the onion to the skillet and sauté until it is translucent. Add the garlic to the skillet.
5. Once the garlic and the onions have cooked, add the kale leaves.
6. Sauté on a medium flame and stir occasionally. You have to ensure that you are turning the leaves over to cook them well. This will mix the onion and the bacon well.
7. Cook the kale until it is softened. This may take an hour.

Grain less Pesto Mozzarella fried Pizza

Serves 2

Ingredients:
- 2 tablespoon garlic infused olive oil
- 2/3 cup tomato sauce
- 3 cups mozzarella cheese
- Parmesan cheese, grated, to taste
- Italian seasoning to taste

Toppings:
- 4 tablespoons pesto
- ½ cup mozzarella cheese, grated
- 4 small mozzarella balls, sliced into 8 slices

Method:
1. Place a nonstick pan with garlic oil over medium heat. When the oil is heated, add mozzarella. Stir with a spatula and spread it all over the pan.
2. When it starts browning around the edges, spread tomato sauce over it. Cook for a minute.
3. Lift the pizza gently with a spatula and place in a lined baking dish.
4. Sprinkle Parmesan cheese and seasoning. Sprinkle mozzarella over it. Drizzle pesto. Place mozzarella slices.
5. Broil in a preheated oven for 2 minutes.
6. Slices into wedges and serve.

Herb Baked Salmon

Serves: 3

Ingredients
- 1 pound salmon fillets
- 2 ounces sesame oil
- ¼ cup tamari soy sauce
- ½ tsp. garlic (minced)
- ¼ tsp. ginger (ground)
- ¼ tsp. basil
- ½ tsp. oregano leaves
- ¼ tsp. thyme
- ¼ tsp. rosemary
- ¼ tsp. tarragon
- 2 ounces butter
- ¼ cup fresh mushrooms (chopped)
- ¼ cup green onions (chopped)

Method

1. Cut the salmon fillets to fill one cup.
2. Take a small plastic bag and place the salmon in the bag. Leave it in the deep freeze.
3. Mix the sauce, the oil and the spices together.
4. Add this mixture to the salmon and place the salmon back into the refrigerator. Leave it to marinate for a few hours.
5. Preheat the oven to 300 degrees Fahrenheit.
6. Take a baking tray and line it with foil.
7. Take the salmon out of the deep freeze and place it in the pan. Make sure that the salmon is all in one layer.
8. Bake the salmon fillets for 15 – 20 minutes.
9. While the salmon is baking, you will need to start cooking the vegetables.
10. Take a small bowl and add the vegetables to it. Melt the butter and add the butter to the bowl. Make sure that all the vegetables are coated well with the butter.
11. Remove the pan from the oven and add the butter and vegetable mixture to the pan.
12. Leave the pan back in the oven for fifteen minutes. Serve it hot!

Sweet & Salt cured Salmon with Scrambled Eggs and Chives

Serves 2

Ingredients:
- 4 eggs
- 7 tablespoons whipping cream
- 4 tablespoons butter
- 2 tablespoon chopped fresh chives
- 2- 6 slices of cured salmon
- Salt & pepper to taste

Method:
1. Beat eggs. Put the pan on medium heat to melt the butter, and add beaten eggs into it. Keep stirring and add cream into it.
2. Reduce the heat and keep stirring the mixture until it becomes creamy.
3. Garnish it with chopped chives, salt & pepper, and serve it with slices of cured salmon.

Stuffed Poblano Peppers

Serves: 4

Ingredients:
- 2 pounds ground pork
- 8 poblano peppers
- 2 vine tomatoes, diced
- 1 small onion, sliced
- 2 tablespoons bacon fat
- 14 baby portabella mushrooms, sliced
- 1/2 cup cilantro, chopped
- Salt to taste
- Pepper powder to taste
- 2 teaspoons chili powder or to taste
- 2 teaspoons cumin powder
- 2 cloves garlic, minced

Method:

1. Set the oven on broil. Place poblano peppers on a cookie sheet and broil in the oven for 8-10 minutes until charred. Turn them around every couple of minutes.
2. Peel the outer skin of the poblano peppers.
3. Place a pan over medium high heat. Add bacon fat, pork, salt and pepper. Cook until brown. Add cumin powder and chili powder.
4. Remove the pork from the pan set it aside. Add onions and garlic to the pan and sauté until translucent. Add mushrooms and sauté for a while. Add tomatoes and cilantro.
5. Make a long slit in the poblano pepper from the start of the stem to bottom of the pepper. Deseed the peppers.
6. Stuff the pork mixture into the peppers. Bake at 350 degrees F for about 8 minutes.
7. Remove from oven and serve.

Shrimp chow mein

Serves: 4

Ingredients
- 1 medium spaghetti squash
- 1 large cup shrimp, deveined & peeled
- 4 small cups slaw mix
- 2 green onions, thinly sliced
- 2 minced garlic cloves
- 2 dried red peppers
- ½ teaspoon minced ginger
- 1 teaspoon whole pepper corns
- 1 tablespoon sesame oil
- 3 tablespoon coconut aminos
- ¾ teaspoon salt
- 1 tablespoon palm sugar

Method
1. Preheat the oven to 300 degrees F.
2. Slice the squash into two halves and bake for about 40 minutes. Once it cools down, add it to a spiralizer and make thin noodles out of it.
3. Heat some sesame oil in a saucepan over medium heat.
4. Add minced garlic, green onion, ginger, red peppers, peppercorn and fry for about 2 minutes until the ingredients start releasing their fragrance.
5. Now add the shrimp, some salt, sugar and cook for about 4-5 minutes until it the shrimp turns tender.
6. Slide in the slaw mix and cook for another 2 minutes until turns soft.
7. Now add the spaghetti noodles and toss well. Remove from flame and transfer on to a large plate.
8. Sprinkle the coconut aminos on top and serve hot.

Mushrooms Burgers

Serves: 2

Ingredients:

For the bun:
- 4 Portobello mushroom caps
- 1 tablespoon extra-virgin coconut oil
- 2 cloves garlic
- 2 teaspoon oregano
- Salt to taste & freshly ground pepper to taste

For the patty:
- 12 ounce beef, ground
- 2 tablespoon Dijon mustard
- Salt to taste
- Freshly ground black pepper to taste
- ½ cup cheddar cheese

Method:
1. Mix together in a bowl, coconut oil, garlic, oregano, salt, and pepper.
2. Clean the Portobello mushrooms and add it to the bowl to marinate.
3. Meanwhile heat a griddle on high flame and grill the mushrooms.
4. In another bowl, mix together beef, Dijon mustard, salt, pepper, and cheese.
5. Mix together and shape into 2 patties. Grill the patties.
6. Place a patty in between 2 mushroom caps to make a burger. Serve with onions and tomatoes.

No Grain Cheese Pizza Rolls

Serves 2:

Ingredients:
- ½ cup chopped red & green peppers
- 2 tablespoon chopped onions
- 2 cups mozzarella cheese
- ½ cup sausages, cooked & crumbled
- 1 teaspoon pizza seasoning
- ¼ cup pizza sauce
- 1 -2 grape tomatoes, sliced

Method:
1. Place a large parchment paper in a baking pan and grease it lightly with olive oil
2. Spread the grated cheese evenly in the baking pan without any gaps.
3. Season it with pizza seasoning.
4. Put it in the preheated oven to and bake at 400 degrees F it until cheese turn brown and gets fully baked.
5. Take out from the oven and gently remove from the baking pan.
6. Garnish the cheese base with crumbled sausages, diced onions, red & green peppers and sliced tomatoes.
7. Top up with tomato sauce and sprinkle more pizza seasoning over it.
8. Place it back in the oven for 10 more minutes, until it gets baked evenly on all sides.
9. Take out the pizza and cut it into thick stripes and roll it up, serve when it gets set.

Keto Meatloaf

Ingredients

- 4 tsp. Dijon mustard
- 2 pound Italian sausage
- 4 tbsp. butter for sautéing
- 4 pounds 85% ground beef
- 1 cup almond flour
- 2 tbsp. thyme leaves*
- ½ cup minced fresh parsley leaves*
- 1 cup shredded Parmesan cheese (not dry grated)
- 4 T Ellen's Low Carb Barbecue sauce
- ½ cup heavy cream
- 12 ounces of cream cheese
- 4 eggs
- 2 tbsp. fresh basil leaves, chopped fine*
- 4 cups shredded cheddar cheese
- 2 cups chopped green pepper
- 12 ounces chopped white onion
- 2 tsp. salt
- ¼ tsp. unflavored gelatin
- 1 tsp. ground black pepper
- 8 garlic cloves, minced

Method:

1. Preheat the oven to 300 degrees Fahrenheit.
2. Take a glass baking-dish and grease it with butter.
3. In a small bowl add the Parmesan cheese and almond flour and mix it well together.
4. Take another bowl and add the softened cheese and the cheddar cheese and mix together. Stir it well so that the mixture becomes smooth and be spread over bread without any lumps.
5. Heat a saucepan over a medium flame. When the pan gets hot, pour the oil in the pan, once it is warmed, add the onion, garlic and pepper to the pan and sauté well. Cook all the ingredients until the onions become translucent and soft.
6. Once done, remove the saucepan from the flame and let the ingredients cool.
7. Once the onion garlic mix has cooled, blend them in a food processor.
8. In another small bowl, whisk the eggs well until there are no bubbles in the bowl. Toss the spices in the egg mixture and season with salt, pepper and the barbecue sauce. Mix it all well.
9. Once all the ingredients have incorporated well, add the cream and mix.
10. When it all mixes well, sprinkle the gelatin and let it set for ten minutes.
11. While that is getting set, chop the beef and Italian sausage finely. Once they are chopped, mix them well. They need to have a mince like consistency and you shouldn't be able to tell the meat apart from the flour.
12. Ensure that the mixture does not stick too much. If it is sticky, add the Parmesan cheese as required, one spoon at a time!
13. Knead the mixture well until it become soft.

14. Next up, mix the meatloaf mixture with the egg mixture. Stir it well and then add all the other ingredients to this mixture. If you want, you can add one ingredient at a time or all together – just ensure that every ingredient gets mixed well.
15. Do not add in the flour at once, keep adding the flour one spoon at a time and continue to mix well. Once you feel that all the ingredients have mixed well, you can stop the kneading.
16. Take a cookie sheet and grease it with butter, cooking spray or oil. Keep the meat mixture on this sheet and allow it to rest. Once done, add the cream and the cheese mixture on the meat. Ensure that you cover the meat with the cream and cheese mixture well.
17. When the meat is covered, roll the cookie sheet from one end with the meat so that the meat layer covers the cream and cheese mixture. Remove the paper off the sheet once done.
18. Seal the ends of the meat roll so that the cheese and the cream stay in and don't ooze out.
19. Take a baking tray and grease it well. Carefully keep the meat roll on the tray and bake it for 15 minutes.
20. Ensure that the meat is well cooked. You can do so by inserting a food thermometer in the meat, the meat has to be 300 degrees Fahrenheit.
21. Let it cool when done.
22. Serve the loaf with sauce!

Tuna curry

Ingredients
- 1 cup tuna, chopped
- 1/2 cup walnuts, chopped
- 1/4 cup almonds, chopped
- 2 hardboiled eggs
- 2 tablespoons low carb mayo
- Salt to taste
- Chili powder to taste
- 1 tablespoon curry powder
- Parsley to sprinkle

Method
1. Start by adding the oil to a pan and add in the walnuts and almonds.
2. Once it browns, add the curry powder, salt and chili powder and give it a good mix.
3. Once it browns, add in the chopped tuna.
4. Add in enough water and cover it.
5. Once it cooks, ladle it into a bowl.
6. Place the boiled eggs on top and spoon over it some of the mayo.
7. Serve hot with cauliflower rice.

Beef stew and leeks

Ingredients:
- 1 pound ground beef
- 2 cups chopped leeks
- 2 cups diced carrots
- 2 cups chopped onions
- 1 tsp. dried sage
- 1 cup chopped beans
- 1 cup chopped tomatoes
- 1 cup chopped mushrooms
- 1 cup chopped zucchini
- 1 cup cubed sweet potato
- 1 tsp. oregano
- 1 tbsp. olive oil
- 3 cups water
- Salt and pepper to taste

Method:
1. Add oil to a skillet placed on medium flame and sauté the onions until they have turned golden brown.
2. Add the ground beef to the pan and cook until the beef has browned.
3. Now, add the remaining ingredients to the pan and continue to cook until you obtain a thick mixture.
4. Add the leeks to the pan and continue to cook until they have softened.
5. When the ingredients start to boil, cover the pan and simmer for a while.
6. Serve hot.

Pizza with Sausages

Ingredients

- 2 tbsp. olive oil
- 1 cauliflower head (trim and then chop the head into smaller pieces)
- 1 ounce white onion (minced)
- 3 tbsp. butter
- ½ cup water
- 4 eggs (2 large eggs)
- 3 cups mozzarella cheese (shredded and chopped into smaller pieces)
- 2 tsp. fennel seeds
- 3 tsp. Italian seasoning
- ½ cup parmesan (grated)
- 5 ounces Pizza Sauce (pick a sauce that is very low in carbohydrates)
- 1 pound Italian sausage (look for the sausage that has a very low amount of carbohydrates)
- 1 cup Italian cheese (preferably get the five cheese blend. You will have to shred the cheese.)

Method

For the crust

1. Preheat the oven to 400 degrees Fahrenheit.
2. Take a cookie sheet and grease it well with the olive oil.
3. Take a large skillet and place it on a medium flame.
4. Add the butter to the skillet and add the onions to the skillet and sauté them until they are translucent. Add the cauliflower to the skillet and cook it until it is almost done.
5. Add water to the skillet and cover the skillet. Leave the vegetables in until the cauliflower is cooked and soft.
6. Transfer the vegetables to a glass bowl and leave them to cool.
7. As the cauliflower is cooling, you will need to cook the Italian sausages. You will need to break them into smaller pieces and cook them well. Drain all the fat out from the skillet. Pat the sausages dry on a tissue paper to remove any excess fat. Leave these aside to cool.
8. Once the cauliflower has cooled down, take three cups of the cauliflower and place it in a food processor or a blender. You will need to blend it until the cauliflower has turned into a smooth puree. Move the puree into a mixing bowl.
9. Add the eggs to the mixing bowl along with the cheese and the spices. Blend them well. Now add the Parmesan cheese and mix it well!
10. Add the cauliflower puree to the cookie sheet and spread it neatly with a spatula. You will have to have a certain thickness all around the sheet.
11. Bake the crust in the oven for twenty minutes. Remove the crust when you find that it has turned brown at the edges.

12. While the pizza crust is in the oven, you will need to chop the sausages into fine pieces. You could either cut the sausage or process it in the food processor.
13. Pour the pizza sauce in a saucepan and add the Italian sausage to the pan.
14. Cook the sausage in the pizza sauce until the sauce has become thick.

For the pizza
1. Once the crust is cooked, you can remove it from the oven and turn the oven settings to boil. Leave the oven shelf four inches from the broiler.
2. Pour the sausage and sauce mixture over the crust. Spread the mixture over the crust using a spatula. You will have a thin coating of the sauce and the sausage. You could add more sausage and sauce to the crust if you want.
3. Leave the pizza in the oven and broil it until the cheese melts. You have to ensure that the cheese has begun to bubble.
4. Remove the pizza from the oven and cut how many ever slices you want.

Bacon Chuck Roast Stew

Serves: 4 to 5

Ingredients
- 1 cup bacon strips
- 3 pounds chuck roast, fat trimmed
- 2 large red onions, sliced
- 2 minced garlic cloves
- 1 ½ teaspoon sea salt
- 1 teaspoon freshly ground black pepper
- 5 cups beef broth
- 1 teaspoon thyme
- 1 tablespoon olive oil
- Some chopped parsley for garnish

Method
1. Using a sharp knife, slice up the roast into thin pieces or small 2-inch chunks.
2. Heat tablespoon of olive oil over medium heat in a large saucepan.
3. Add the onion slices to it and sauté for 3 to 4 minutes until they start releasing water.
4. Now add the minced garlic and cook for another minute.
5. Pour some beef broth into the pan and sprinkle some salt, thyme and pepper on top. Stir all the ingredients well using a large wooden spoon.
6. Slide in the chuck roast chunks, bacon slices and cover the pan with a lid. Cook the stew for about 90 minutes on high flame and then let it simmer for another 15-20 minutes. If you are using a slow cooker, cook on low heat for 7 hours until the roast is completely cooked.
7. Transfer in a large plate and garnish with some chopped parsley on top.
8. Serve hot.

Chicken Guadalajara

Ingredients
- 4 tbsp. butter
- 8 ounces white onions (chopped finely)
- 6 garlics (minced cloves)
- 8 boneless, skinless, chicken breast halves
- 6 ounces cans diced tomatoes
- 6 ounces cans of green chilies
- 1 cup whipped cream
- 1 cup chicken broth
- 1 tsp. cayenne pepper
- 1 tsp. cumin (dried)
- 1 tsp. garlic powder
- 2 tsp. sea salt
- Grated cheddar cheese (garnish)
- Sour cream (garnish)
- Salsa (garnish)

Method

1. Wash the chicken breasts and pat them dry. Cut them into slices.

2. Take a medium sized skillet and place it on a medium flame. Melt the butter in the skillet and add the onions and garlic to the skillet. Cook them until the onions are soft.

3. Add the chicken to the skillet and cook it well. Drain out all the fat from the chicken.

4. Reduce the heat and add the tomatoes and the chili to the skillet.

5. Cover the skillet and continue to cook it for another fifteen minutes.

6. Add the cream cheese to the skillet and stir until the cheese has melted well. Add the sour cream and mix well.

7. You will have to ensure that the chicken and the vegetables were coated well with cheese.

8. Add the broth to the sauce and mix well.

9. Top with garnishes and serve hot

Simple beef stew

Ingredients
- 2 lbs. beef
- 5 cups beef broth
- Salt to taste
- Pepper to taste
- 1 teaspoon chili powder
- 1 teaspoon Worcestershire sauce
- 2 tablespoons olive oil
- 1 red onion, chopped
- 2 tablespoon garlic, chopped
- 3 medium carrots
- 4 medium celery sticks

Method
1. Start by add in the beef to a bowl and add the salt, pepper and chili powder to it.
2. Mix it until well combined.
3. Add the Worcestershire sauce to it and mix.
4. Set it aside.
5. Meanwhile, add the oil to a pan and allow it to heat.
6. Add in the garlic and brown it.
7. Add the onion, carrots and celery sticks.
8. Add the beef stock and allow it to come to a boil.
9. Add in the beef and wait for it to boil.
10. Cover with a lid and simmer it.
11. You must cook it for 1 to 2 hours or until the meat is completely cooked.

Lemon Rosemary Chicken Thighs

Ingredients:
- 6 chicken thighs
- 1 1/2 lemons
- 3 cloves garlic
- 6 sprigs rosemary
- Salt to taste
- Pepper powder to taste
- 3 tablespoons butter

Method:
1. Sprinkle chicken with salt and pepper.
2. Place a cast iron skillet over high heat. Place chicken thighs over the skillet. With its skin side down and cook until brown. Flip sides and brown the other side too. Sprinkle a little lemon juice over it. Chop the remaining lemon and add it to the pan and sauté.
3. Add garlic and rosemary and sauté.
4. Transfer the skillet into a preheated oven and bake at 400 degrees F for about 30 minutes.
5. Remove from oven and add butter and bake until crisp. Discard the lemon pieces.
6. Serve with sautéed vegetables.

Chapter 7: Dessert Recipes

Baked Ricotta Custard

Ingredients:
- 2 large egg whites
- 2 large eggs
- 1/2 cup half and half
- 1 1/2 cups ricotta cheese
- 1/4 cup erythritol or to taste
- 1/2 teaspoon vanilla extract
- 2 tablespoons ground cinnamon

Method:
1. Add ricotta and cream cheese to the mixing bowl and beat with an electric mixer until smooth and creamy.
2. Add erythritol and beat until well blended.
3. Add remaining ingredients and beat until well blended.
4. Transfer into 8 ramekins. Take a large baking dish. Pour enough hot water to cover 1 inch from the bottom of the dish.
5. Place the ramekins inside the baking dish.
6. Bake in a preheated oven at 250 degrees F for about 45 minutes or until set.
7. Remove from the oven and cool.
8. Sprinkle cinnamon.
9. Serve either chilled or at room temperature.

Chocolate Cake in a Mug

Serves: 2

Ingredients:
- 2 eggs, beaten
- 4 tablespoons cocoa powder
- 4 tablespoons sugar substitute of choice or to taste
- A pinch salt
- 2 tablespoons heavy cream
- 1 teaspoon vanilla extract
- ½ teaspoon baking powder
- Cooking spray
- Whipped cream to serve
- Berries of your choice to serve

Method:
1. Mix together cocoa, sweetener, salt and baking powder in a bowl.
2. Add cream, vanilla, and egg and mix well.
3. Pour into mugs greased with cooking spray. (½ fill it)
4. Microwave on high for about 60-80 seconds until the top of the cake is slightly hard.
5. Cool and invert on to a plate. Serve with whipped cream and berries.

Coconut Cream Macaroons

Ingredients:
- 4 eggs whites
- 16 ounces dried coconut (unsweetened, dried and finely shredded)
- 1 tsp. vanilla
- 8 ounces cream cheese (soften at room temperature)
- ½ tsp. cream of tartar
- 2 ounce Sugar free white chocolate syrup
- 2 cup erythritol
- 2 ounce heavy cream
- 2 ounce chocolate chips
- 1/4 tsp. salt

Method:
1. Preheat the oven to 300 degrees Fahrenheit.
2. Take a cookie sheet and line it with parchment paper.
3. Take a large mixing bowl and beat the egg whites, the cream of tartar and the salt using an electric mixer or a blender.
4. Add the erythritol only one tablespoon at a time and keep beating the mixture until the mixture is smooth.
5. Add the coconut and keep folding it well.
6. Add the cream cheese and the heavy cream and smoothen the mixture. Add the syrup and mix the ingredients well.
7. Add the coconut mixture in thirds until it has combined well. Add the chocolate chips and fold the dough well.
8. Use a small scoop and add the coconut mixture to the sheet.
9. Leave them in the oven to cook for thirty minutes. Once they have been cooked for that long, leave them in the oven to dry for another thirty minutes.
10. Transfer back to the rack to cool.

Brownie Cheesecake

Ingredients:
For brownie base:
- 1 large egg, beaten
- 1/4 cup butter
- 2 tablespoons cocoa powder, unsweetened
- 1 ounce chocolate, chopped
- 1/4 cup almond flour
- A pinch salt
- 6 tablespoons granulated erythritol or Swerve sweetener
- 2 tablespoons walnuts or pecans, chopped
- 1/4 teaspoon vanilla

For cheesecake filling
- 1 large egg
- 1/4 cup granulated erythritol or Swerve sweetener
- 1/2 pound cream cheese, softened
- 1/4 teaspoon vanilla extract
- 2 tablespoons heavy cream

Method:

1. Line a small spring form pan with aluminum foil.
2. Add butter and chocolate to a microwave safe bowl and microwave for about a minute or until the chocolate melts.
3. Remove from the microwave and whisk well.
4. Mix together almond flour, cocoa and salt in a bowl.
5. To the beaten egg, add sweetener add vanilla and whisk until smooth. Add almond flour mixture and whisk well.
6. Add melted chocolate mixture and whisk until smooth.
7. Add nuts and stir. Transfer this mixture into the lined baking dish.
8. Bake in a preheated oven at 325°F for about 15 minutes. The center should be soft and edges should be set.
9. Remove from the oven and cool. Place crust on a baking sheet along with the baking dish.
10. Meanwhile, make the filling as follows: Add cream cheese to a bowl and beat until smooth. Add eggs, Swerve, cream, and vanilla and beat until well combined.
11. Transfer the filling over the baked crust and spread it.
12. Place the baking sheet in the oven and bake for another 35-40 minutes.
13. When it is cooled, loosen the edges of the crust with a sharp knife and place on a plate.
14. Cover with cling wrap. Chill and serve later.

Strawberry Swirl Ice cream

Ingredients:
For vanilla ice cream:
- 2 cups heavy cream
- 2 tablespoons vodka (optional)
- 6 large egg yolks
- 2/3 cup erythritol
- 1/4 teaspoon xanthan gum (optional)
- 1 teaspoon vanilla extract

For strawberry swirl ice cream:
- 2 cups strawberries, pureed

Method:
1. Place a heavy bottomed pan over low heat. Add cream and erythritol. Heat until erythritol dissolves. Remove from heat.
2. Add eggs to the mixing bowl and beat with an electric mixer until it doubles in volume.
3. Add about 2 tablespoons of the warm cream to the egg and beat constantly. Repeat this procedure until all the cream is added. Add vanilla and beat again.
4. Add vodka and xanthan gum if using and beat again. Cool completely.
5. Freeze the ice cream for a couple of hours. Stir in between a couple of times while it is being frozen.
6. Remove the semi-frozen ice cream from the freezer.
7. Swirl the strawberry puree all around on the top. With a knife, lightly mix to get a ripple effect.
8. Freeze the ice cream for another 5-6 hours or until set. Remove from the freezer around 30 minutes before serving.
9. Alternately, you can freeze in an ice cream maker following the manufacturer's instructions. Then follow steps 7 and 8. Add strawberry puree during the last few minutes of churning.
10. For making vanilla ice cream, omit steps 6 and 7. Freeze until set.

Keto Pound Cake

Ingredients:
- 10 eggs
- 2 cups butter
- 4 cups hazelnut flour
- 2 teaspoons vanilla extract
- 2 teaspoons baking powder
- 2 teaspoons Stevia
- A pinch of salt

Method:
1. Add all the dry ingredients to a bowl.
2. Add cream and sweetener to a mixing bowl. Beat with an electric mixer until creamy.
3. Add an egg at a time and beat each time.
4. Add about 2 tablespoons of the dry mixture to the mixing bowl and beat each time. Continue until all the dry mixture is added.
5. Add vanilla extract and beat again.
6. Pour into a greased and lined baking dish.
7. Bake in a preheated oven 350°F for about 40-50 minutes or until a toothpick when inserted comes out clean.

Lemon Meringue Tartlets

Serves: 4

Ingredients:

For lemon curd:
- 6 egg yolks
- 20 drops liquid Stevia
- 7 tablespoons butter, cubed
- ½ cup powdered erythritol
- 1 large pinch xanthan gum
- 4 lemons

For crust:
- 2 cups almond flour
- 1 egg
- 4 tablespoons whey protein
- 2 tablespoons butter, melted
- 4 tablespoons powdered erythritol
- ½ teaspoon salt

For Meringue:
- 4 egg whites
- 4 tablespoons powdered erythritol
- ¼ teaspoon cream of tartar

Method:
1. Preheat oven to 350F.
2. To make crust: Add all the ingredients of the crust into a bowl and mix with your hands to form dough.
3. Divide the dough into 4 portions and place in tartlet pans. Press it into the pan.
4. Bake in preheated oven at 350F for about 10-15 minutes. Check every 5 minutes. Remove it if it is done.
5. To make lemon curd: Grate the rind of 2 lemons into a bowl. Also squeeze the juice of the zested lemons into the bowl.
6. Whisk the yolks in a heatproof bowl. Add Stevia drops and erythritol. Whisk well. Place the bowl in a double boiler. Whisk until it becomes slightly thick.
7. Add remaining lemon juice and lemon zest and whisk again. Add xanthan. Whisk.
8. Add butter cubes, one at a time and whisk each time until it melts. Continue doing this until all the butter cubes are added.
9. Remove the bowl from the double boiler and place in the refrigerator for a few hours to chill.
10. For meringue: Add whites into a bowl and beat with an electric mixer on low speed until it is frothy in texture.
11. Add cream of tartar and beat. Now increase the speed of the mixer to medium. Add erythritol, a tablespoon at a time. Add cream of tartar and beat again.
12. Increase the speed of mixer to high speed. Beat until stiff peaks are formed.
13. To assemble tartlets: Divide the lemon curd and spoon into the prepared crust.
14. Spoon some meringue over it.
15. Bake at 350 degrees F for 20 minutes or until golden.

Strawberry Shortcakes

Ingredients:

For shortcakes:

- 6 ounces cream cheese
- 4 tablespoons erythritol
- 6 large eggs, separated
- 1 teaspoon vanilla extract
- 1/2 teaspoon baking powder

For filling:

- 2 cups whipped cream
- 20 medium strawberries, sliced

Method:

1. Beat egg whites until light and fluffy.
2. Add cream cheese to the yolks along with vanilla extract, erythritol, and baking powder. Beat until smooth and creamy.
3. Add whites and fold lightly into the cream cheese mixture.
4. Grease 2-3 large baking sheets. Line with parchment paper or silpat.
5. Drop large spoonfuls on the baking sheet. Leave space between 2 shortcakes.
6. Bake in a preheated oven 300°F for about 25 minutes. You can bake in batches.
7. Spread whipped cream on all the shortcakes. Lay strawberry slices on half the shortcakes. Cover with the remaining shortcakes.

Apple Pie

Ingredients:

<u>For the crust:</u>
- 2 eggs
- 3/4 cup coconut flour
- 1/4 teaspoon salt
- 1/2 cup butter, unsalted (if using salted butter, then omit salt), melted

<u>For filling:</u>
- 3 Macintosh apples, peeled, cored, sliced or chopped
- 2 tablespoons erythritol
- 1/2 teaspoon vanilla extract
- 2 teaspoons ground cinnamon
- 1 tablespoon butter

Method:
1. To make crust: Add butter and eggs to a bowl and whisk until well combined. Add coconut flour and salt and mix again. Finally using your hands, form into dough.
2. Divide the dough into 2 equal parts. Take one part and press into a small pie pan.
3. To make filling: Add apple, erythritol, vanilla and cinnamon to a bowl and toss well.
4. Lay the apple slices on the prepared crust. Arrange it in any manner you desire. Set aside.
5. Take the remaining half of the dough and roll it with a rolling pin on a clean work (dust with a little coconut flour or place over parchment paper) surface to about 1/4 inch thickness.
6. Gently lift the rolled dough and place over the filled crust. Seal the edges by pressing together both the crusts. Using a sharp knife, make slits on the top covering.
7. Alternately, in step 5, after rolling, cut into long strips of about 1 centimeter wide. Place the strips crisscross over the filled crust.
8. Bake in a preheated oven 425°F for about 12 minutes.
9. Lower the temperature to 350°F for about 40 minutes.
10. Remove from the oven and cool for a while.
11. Serve warm with whipped cream or ice cream

Strawberry Basil Ice Cups

Serves: 5

Ingredients:
- 6 tablespoons cream cheese
- 4 tablespoons creamed coconut milk
- 2 tablespoons butter, unsalted, at room temperature
- 2 tablespoons powdered erythritol or Swerve
- Liquid Stevia drops to taste (optional)
- A handful fresh basil leaves
- ½ cup fresh strawberries + extra to garnish
- ½ teaspoon vanilla extract

Method:
1. Add cream cheese, creamed coconut milk, butter, erythritol, Stevia, and vanilla the blender and blend until smooth.
2. Remove half the blended mixture and set aside.
3. To the other half that is in the blender add strawberries and blend until smooth.
4. Divide the mixture into 5 silicone muffin cups.
5. Clean the blender and add the blended mixture that was kept aside. Add basil leaves and blend until smooth.
6. Divide the mixture and spoon into the muffin cups above the strawberry layer.
7. Place thinly sliced strawberry slices on top.
8. Freeze for a few hours until set.

Coconut Cookies

Ingredients:
- White of 1 large egg
- 1/4 cup whole grain soy flour
- 2 tablespoons whole hazelnuts
- 3 tablespoons dried coconut
- 3/4 teaspoon coconut extract
- 4 tablespoons butter, unsalted
- 1-2 tablespoons carbonated water (soda water) or as required
- 1/4 teaspoon vanilla extract
- 4 tablespoons erythritol or Swerve sweetener
- 1/4 teaspoon salt
- Cooking spray

Method:

1. Spread the hazelnuts in a single layer on a baking sheet.
2. Bake in a preheated oven 350°F for about 8-10 minutes or until brown (The skin will be nearly dark brown when done). Remove from the oven and cool.
3. Spread a moist kitchen towel on your work area. Spread the roasted hazelnuts on one half of the towel. Cover with the other half of the towel and rub for a while until the skin peels off.
4. Chop the hazelnuts coarsely and set aside.
5. Add soy flour, coconut, hazelnuts, egg white, carbonated water, coconut extract, vanilla extract, salt, butter and erythritol and mix well.
6. Spray a baking sheet with cooking spray. Place a tablespoon of the batter on the baking sheet. Try to give it a round shape.
7. Bake in a preheated oven 350°F for about 20 minutes or until light golden brown.
8. Remove from the oven and let it cool for a couple of minutes.
9. Transfer onto a wire rack.
10. Cool completely and serve.

Conclusion

With that, we have come to the end of this book. I want to thank you for choosing this book.

Now that you have come to the end of this book, we would first like to express our gratitude for choosing this particular source and taking the time to read through it. All the information here was well researched and put together in a way to help you understand the diet as easily as possible.

The concise manner of describing the diet and providing you with recipes will help you learn all you actually need to know about it. We hope you found it useful and you can now use it as a guide anytime you want. You may also want to recommend it to any family or friends that you think might find it useful as well.

The ketogenic diet is a healthy and easy way to lose weight as well as to get your body into a healthier state than it was before. As we have mentioned in the above chapters, you can see exactly how the diet works and why it will help you. So go ahead and give it a try. We know for sure that you won't regret it.

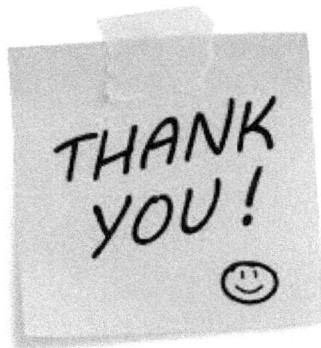

THANK YOU! ☺

Finally, if you enjoyed this book, then I'd like to ask you for a favor, would you be kind enough to leave a review for this book on Amazon? It'd be greatly appreciated!

Click here to leave a review for this book on Amazon!

http://amzn.to/2nheOKs

Thank you and good luck!

www.ingramcontent.com/pod-product-compliance
Lightning Source LLC
Chambersburg PA
CBHW071235020426
42333CB00015B/1478

* 9 7 8 1 9 5 1 1 0 3 6 6 8 *